Feel Better

By Amanda Healan, PhD

I wrote this book for myself.
Now, it is for you.

Consider this book a recovery companion.

This book isn't your doctor

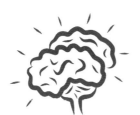

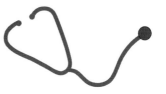

...or your psychiatrist.

Or your concerned friends and family.

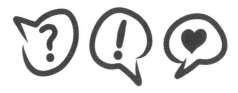

It's a light-hearted place to explore the personal

> "Writing down emotions, thoughts,
> and goals can help you heal."
>   - Science

It doesn't matter what you are recovering from or where you are on your recovery journey. Some recoveries are fast, some are slow. You can start at any time.

Write or draw however you want in this book.

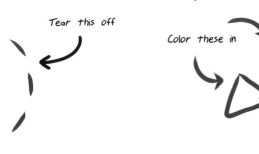

Tear this off

Color these in

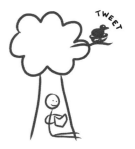

TWEET

You can keep it private like a journal,

or use it as a conversation tool.

Move at your own pace. Take one page a day, take a bunch of pages at once. Take breaks. Go back and revisit pages that click with you. (You can fold down the corners to help with that.)

The simple prompts in this book will help you dig deep, stay focused, and track your progress.

(They may also put a smile on your face.)

In short,

This

book

is designed

to

help

you

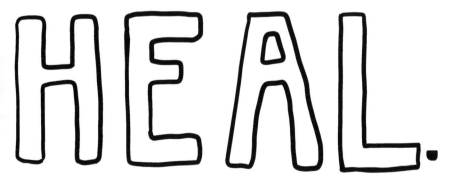

...but before we can begin our recovery,

we need to get in the healing mindset.

Calm.

Quiet.

Peaceful.

Close your eyes and take a few deep breaths.
Take as many as you need.

(Maybe take one more.)

When you're ready,
turn the page to get started.

Nice work!
Let's start with the easy stuff:

HELLO my name is:

EMILY ☺

Pleased to meet you!

Today's date: _____

○ Monday
○ Tuesday
○ Wednesday
○ Thursday
○ Friday
○ Saturday
○ Sunday
○ Who knows?

The weather is:

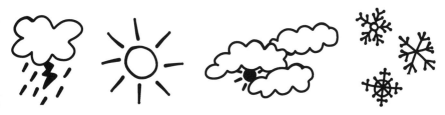

I'm feeling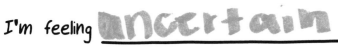

about my recovery.

A drawing of me.

Now let's get to know each other. Understanding who you are, and where you came from, could provide clues to your recovery style.

So, how old are you? How's it been so far?

Age	Interesting event
0	Born
12	first heartbreak
18	engaged ?
19	went to college
?	did some shit
22	graduated college
23	???? help
○	

Who is in your family?

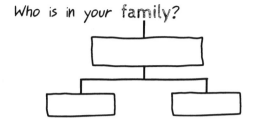

We'll revisit these weirdos later.

I'm an:

Introvert

Extrovert

<u>In the middle</u>-vert

9

Draw some food you like to eat.

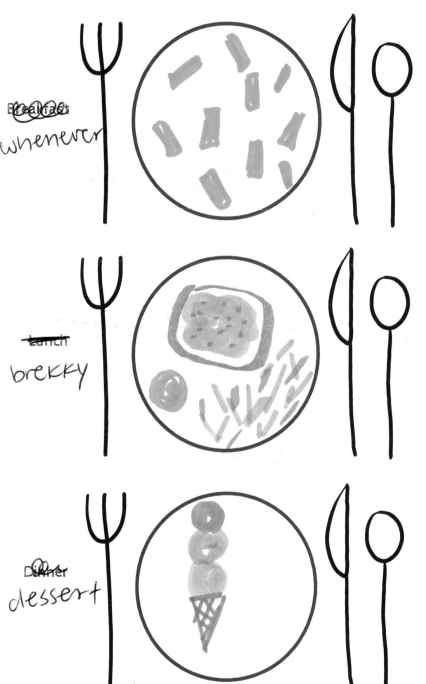

~~Breakfast~~ whenever

~~Lunch~~ brekky

~~Dinner~~ dessert

10

What kind of stuff makes you happy?

my kitty

good food

good coffee

my family

travelling

thrifting

nick

thunderstorms

naps

nostalgia

movies

Write or draw until you've filled the whole page.

Experts agree that a positive attitude can do wonders for a person's recovery. Optimists simply heal faster than pessimists.

You don't have to be a sugar-coated pack of sunshine, but setting healthy, positive expectations for your recovery could be the single largest predictor of success.

Give it a try.
Do you think you can recover? Check all that apply.

- [ ] Certainly
- [ ] Yes
- [ ] Absolutely
- [ ] Without a doubt
- [ ] Of course
- [ ] Indubitably
- [ ] Why not?
- [ ] Surely
- [ ] Yep
- [ ] Quite so
- [ ] By all means
- [ ] DNH _____

Remember:

Attitude and recovery go hand in hand.

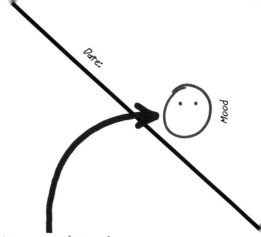

Date:

Mood

Let's add this mood tracker.
Write the date and finish the face,
based on how you're feeling.

Use the tracker to reflect
on your attitude over the
course of your recovery.

14

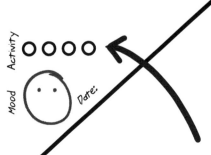

The circles are to track your activity level. Just like a positive attitude, regular exercise can keep you healthy and help you heal. Fill in the circles to match how active you are each day.

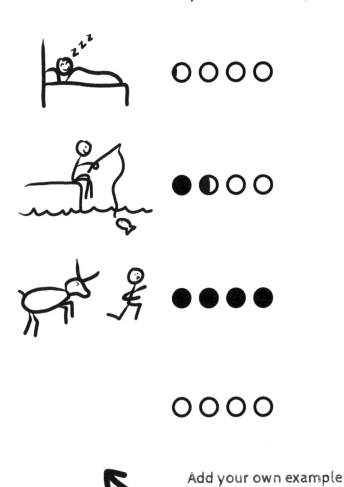

Add your own example

Mood   Activity

It's important to listen to your body to maintain a healthy activity level. You know best when to rest and when to get moving.

Studies (and maybe your own experiences) show too much rest can lead to depression.

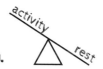

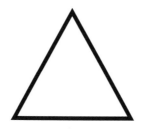
Too much activity leaves no time for healing.

Some people have trouble resting, whlie others struggle to stay active. What is your tendency?

16

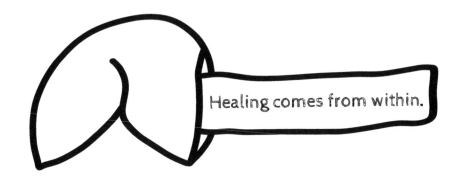

Healing comes from within.

Now that we've gotten to know you a little,
let's get on with the healing.

Everyone has internal factors that contribute to their
recovery. These can include expectations, biases, and
motivations. Some of these factors are clearer than
others. Some are more flexible than others.

Let's explore how these factors relate to you.
(And put some tools in place to help you stay organized.)

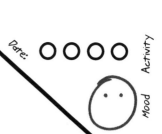
First, expectations.

What will you consider a <u>successful</u> recovery?

Writing out your answers can help you get there.
Putting pen to paper doubles down: first you think about
an idea, then you reinforce it by writing it down.

It's also a little way to put your body into recovery

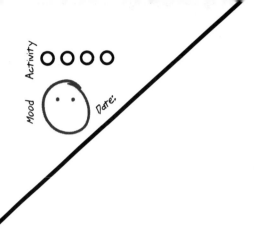

Mood Activity

OOOO

Date:

Next, a tough question.
What might you need to change to recover?

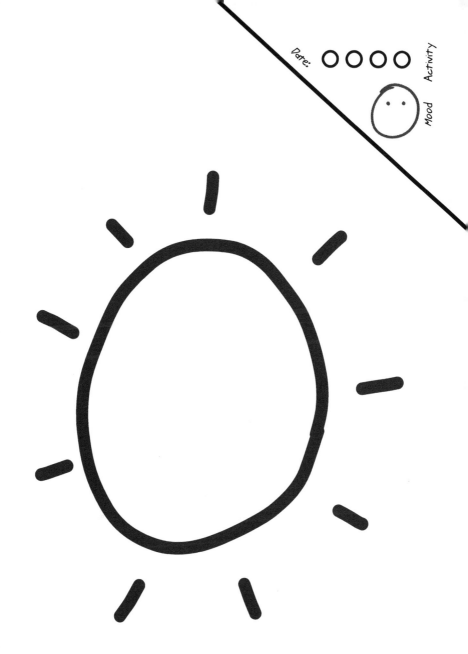

By the way, what are you recovering from?

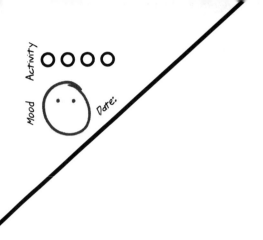

Mood Activity ○○○○ Date:

That sounds complicated.
Can you draw a picture of it instead?

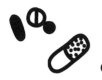

Now we're getting it.
Are there vitamins or medications involved?
Draw them here.

You can also use
the medication log at
the end of this book.

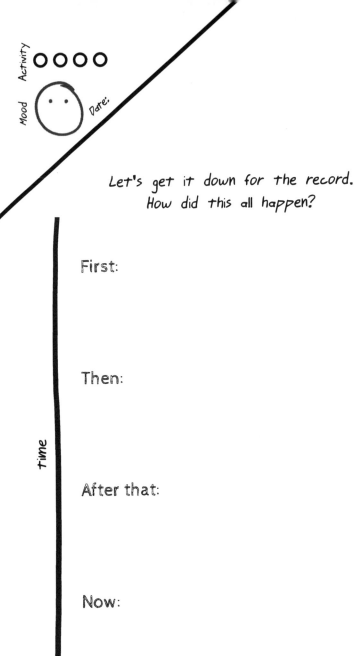

Mood Activity OOOO

Date:

Let's get it down for the record.
How did this all happen?

time

First:

Then:

After that:

Now:

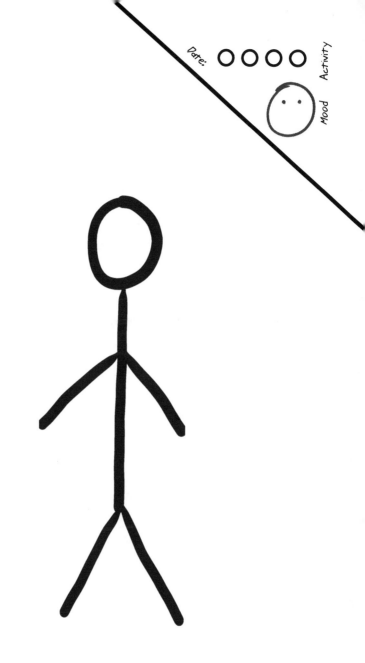

What parts of you need to heal? Point them out.

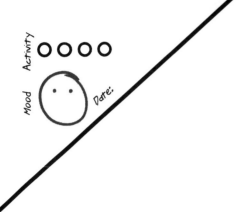

Mood   Activity
○○○○
Date:

You are not alone. Everyone is unique, but you can learn from the experience of others.

Have you talked to anyone who's recovered from the same thing or something similar?

How did it go?

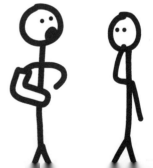

25

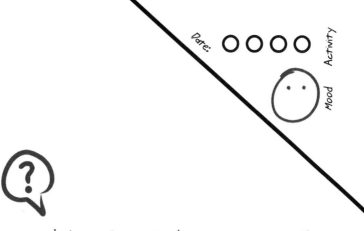

Are there **appointments** involved in your recovery?

Recovery appointments don't have to be formal.
Sometimes you need a doctor,
sometimes you need a good friend.

Humans are social animals! Connecting with others increases
happiness and improves health. It may also help you relieve
stress associated with recovery.

Make plenty of recovery appointments to be sure you feel
supported and well-connected.

Keep track of appointments
using the log at the end of this book.

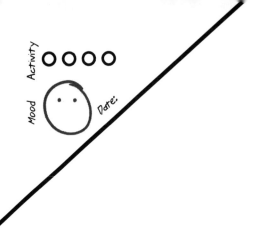

Mood Activity

Date:

You've been working hard. Let's take a fun break.
Draw yourself a treat. Anything you like.

How have people responded
since hearing about all this?
What have people offered?

Write down the names of
as many people as you can think of
who _could_ support you during your recovery.

We get it, they might not.
But put 'em down anyway.

Mood Activity

Date:

Time to check in on your physical health.
How have you been feeling?
Fill in the thermometers.

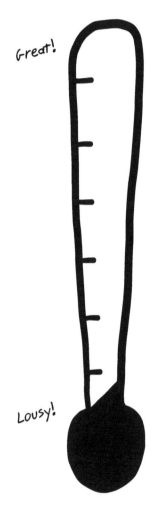

Great!

Lousy!

Last week

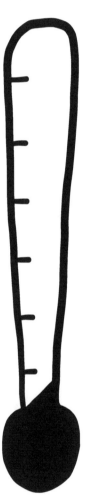

This week

Date: OOOO

We've hinted at this one before, but let's be blunt. Experts say this is perhaps the most important part of any recovery. You'll find it's a recurring theme.

What are your **expectations** for your recovery?

You might want to stop for a while after this page to allow time to reflect. Some pages are like that.

30

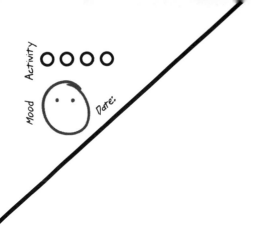
Recovery is tough (nay, impossible) all by yourself.

Whether they know it or not, the people you listed on pages 8, 25, and 28 are part of your recovery team. There might be other team members you can include, like counselors, neighbors, medical professionals, or even pets.

Choose 3 most central to your recovery
and write their names here:

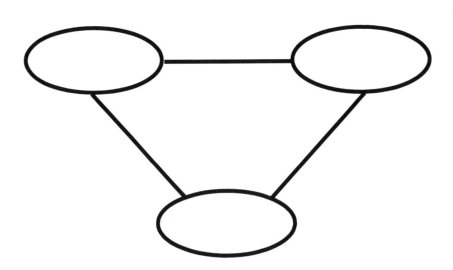

Even with a great team,
you are still in charge of your recovery.
Let's explore your efforts so far.
Jot down any recovery prep you've already done.

PHYSICAL preparations

MENTAL preparations

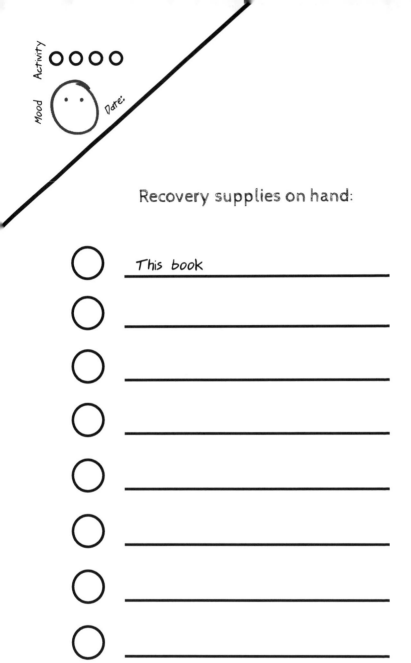

Mood
Activity

O O O O

Date:

Recovery supplies on hand:

O _This book_____

O _____

O _____

O _____

O _____

O _____

O _____

O _____

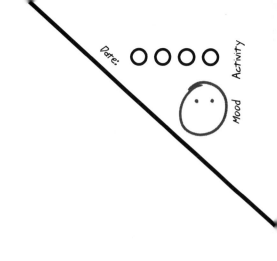

Date: ◯ ◯ ◯ ◯

Mood   Activity

Have you done any research related to your recovery?
What did you find? Any helpful websites or resources?

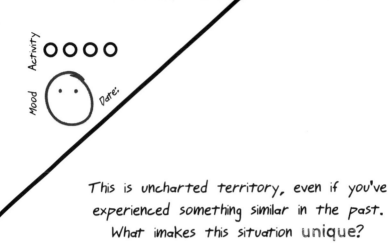

Mood

Activity

Date:

This is uncharted territory, even if you've experienced something similar in the past. What imakes this situation unique?

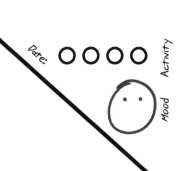

Sounds like you've thought this through. Great!
What do you foresee along your road to recovery?

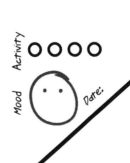

Now dream big both ways.
What is the worst that could happen?

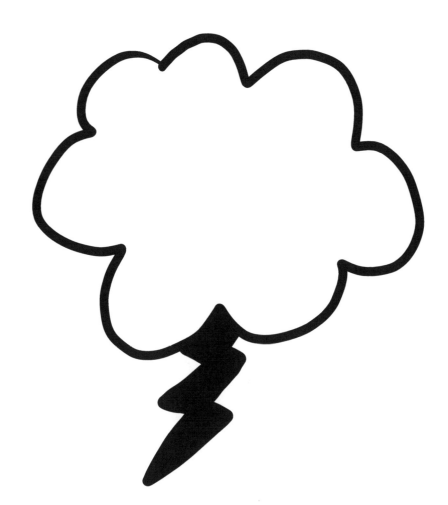

What is the best possible outcome?

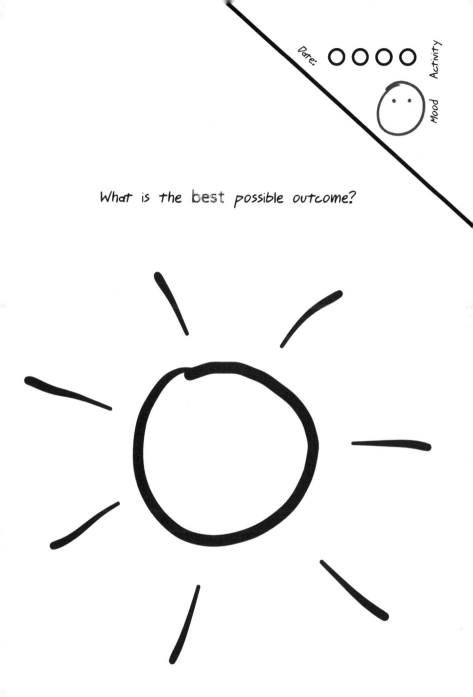

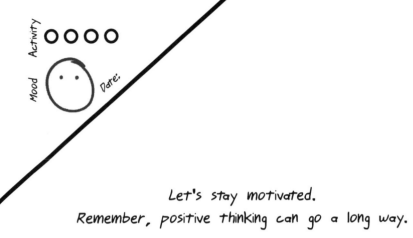

Mood Activity

O O O O

Date:

Let's stay motivated.
Remember, positive thinking can go a long way.

I want to heal because:

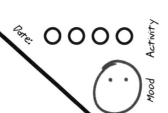
"What is this book? All touchy–feely talk?" —you, maybe.

It's time for action. Time to get something done.
We'll do it together, with help from research that shows
writing down goals helps them happen.

Try it. Set a tiny goal.
We'll check on it in two pages, so keep it simple.
(It can be unrelated to your recovery.)

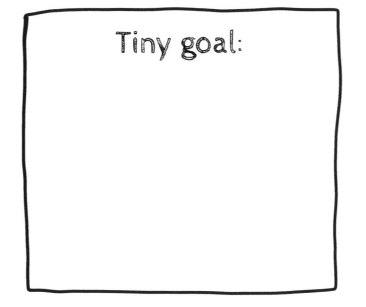

Tiny goal:

Tiny goal ideas: eat a carrot, go outside, call a friend.

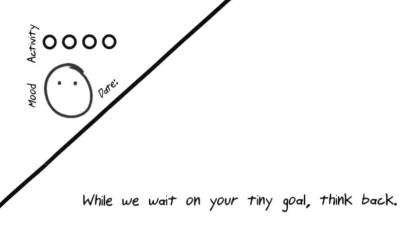

Mood Activity

Date:

While we wait on your tiny goal, think back.

Day 1 (or so) of my recovery went like this:

What has changed since then?

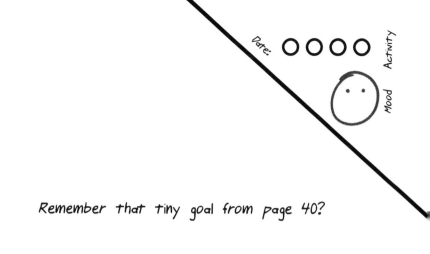

Remember that tiny goal from page 40?

> # Tiny goal results:

If you achieved your goal, way to go!
If not, cross out ~~results~~ and
use the space to set a new one.

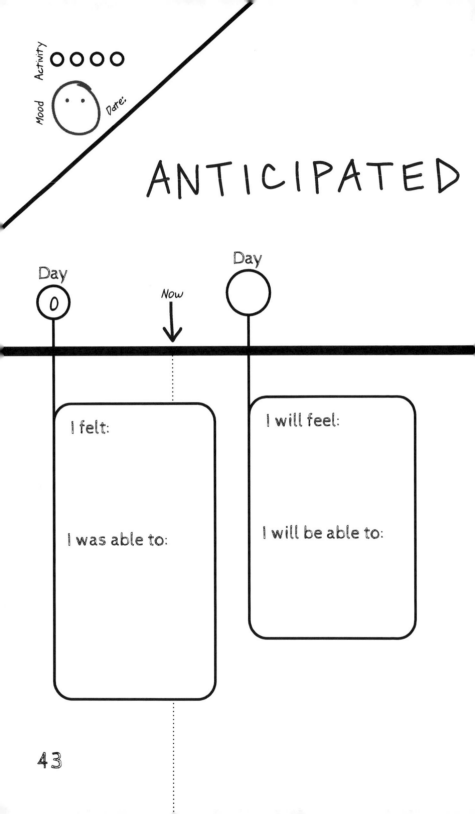

Mood Activity ○○○○ Date:

ANTICIPATED

Day
0

Now

Day

I felt:

I was able to:

I will feel:

I will be able to:

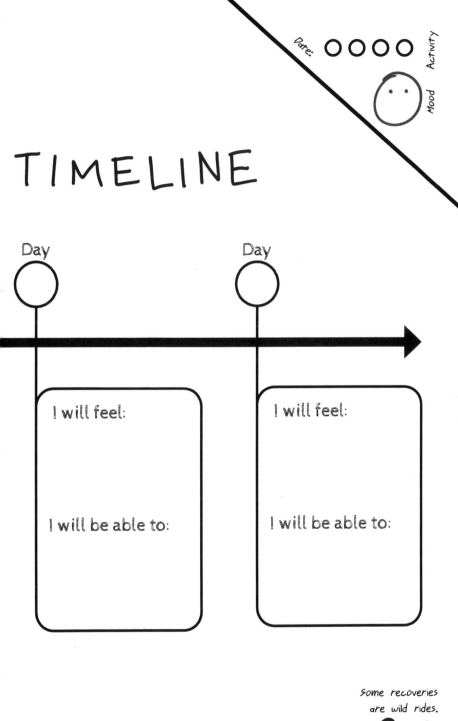

Date: ○○○○

Mood

Activity

TIMELINE

Day

Day

I will feel:

I will be able to:

I will feel:

I will be able to:

Some recoveries
are wild rides.

44

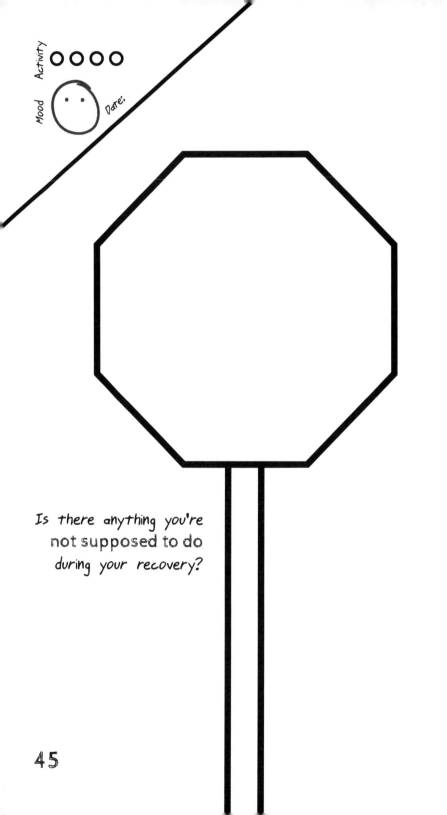

Is there anything you're not supposed to do during your recovery?

Thoughts are powerful.
They can determine your mood.

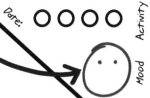

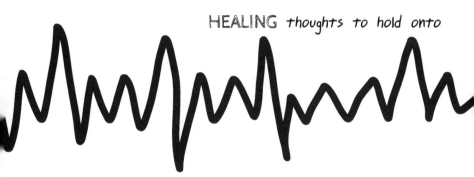

HEALING thoughts to hold onto

WORRYING thoughts I can't shake

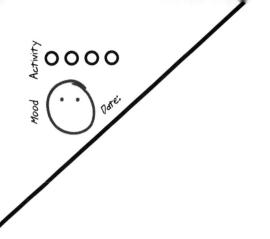

Mood   Activity

Date:

Try this:

Relax your shoulders.

Relax your jaw and tongue.

Breathe in slowly.

Breathe out

slower.

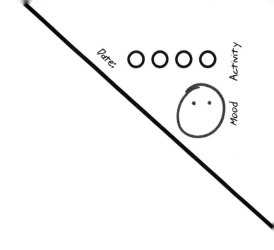

Staying calm can help you heal.

Take a moment to flip back through your mood trackers.
What patterns do you notice?

How is your mood affecting you?

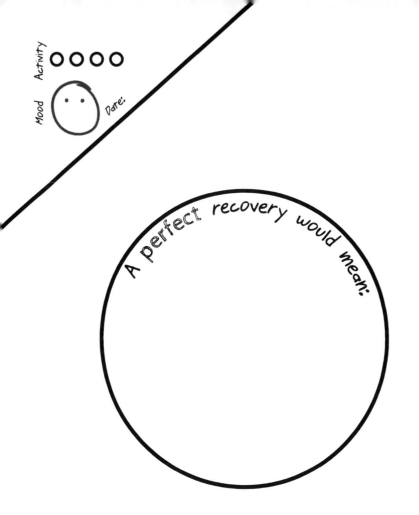

Mood

Activity

○○○○

Date:

A perfect recovery would mean:

Do you expect this outcome?

☐ no

☐ no

49

You've made it quite a ways.
Write an encouraging note to yourself,
tear it out, and put it where you'll see it
first thing tomorrow morning.

Dear _____ ,

You are _____

_____

_____.

With love,

50

Mood Activity O O O O

Date:

You're doing great.
51

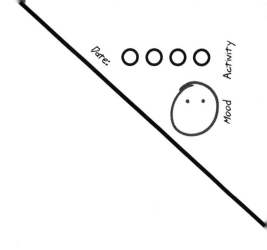

Date: ◯◯◯◯

Activity

Mood

Don't forget, you are always in charge.
This page is for anything you want.
Let something out.

52

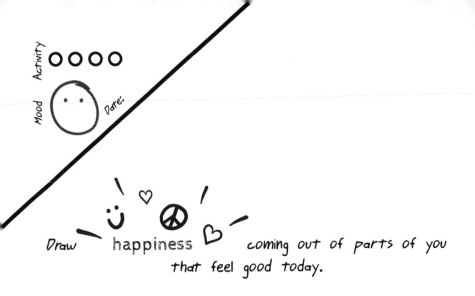

Draw happiness coming out of parts of you that feel good today.

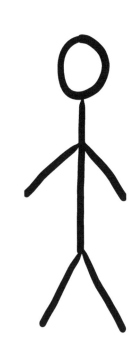

Check in with your body.

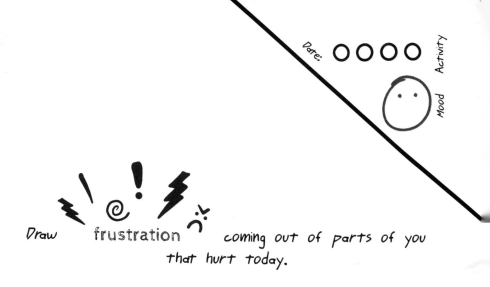

Date: ○ ○ ○ ○

Mood   Activity

Draw **frustration** coming out of parts of you that hurt today.

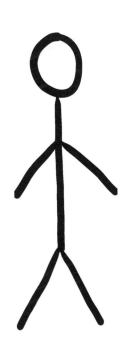

You never know what's stashed inside.

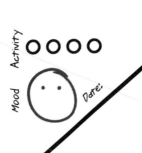

Mood Activity

Date:

Recovery takes stamina.
Remembering your tendencies on page 16,
how full are your tanks? Add arrows to the gauges.

Energy Level

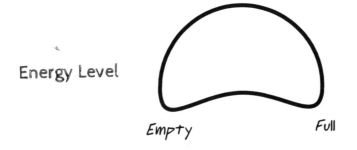

Empty   Full

Motivation Level

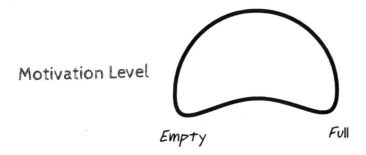

Empty   Full

What can you do to adjust your levels?
Check back on your activity and mood trackers for help.

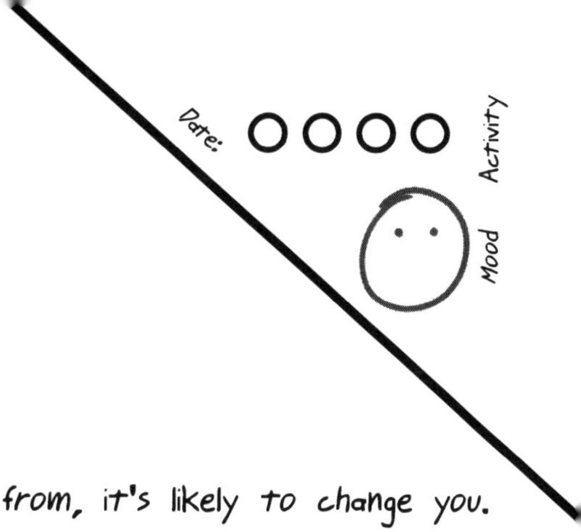

Whatever you are recovering from, it's likely to change you. You might like some changes more than others.

Three things that might be different
when I am fully recovered:

1)

2)

3)

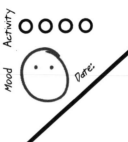
57 No one is watching. Let's talk about hard stuff.
Has anything about your recovery
felt uncomfortable or embarrassing?

Some recoveries require so much energy that they
can make you feel out of the loop or alone.
It's important to stay connected,
even when you are having a hard time.
What's been going on in the world?

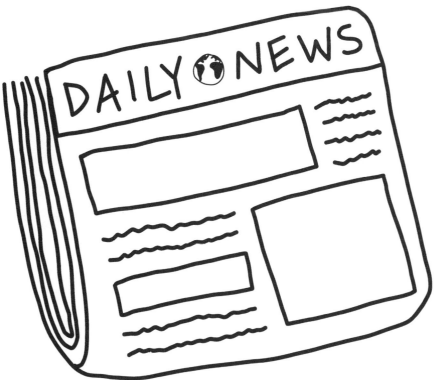

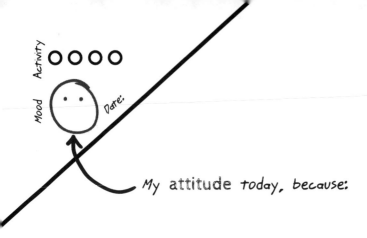

Mood

Activity

O O O O

Date:

My attitude today, because:

Is being mindful of your attitude a priority for you?
Why or why not?

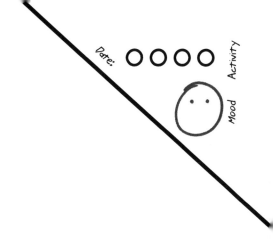

Mood   Activity

No matter your attitude, let's try to make you smile.
(Smiling takes fewer muscles than frowning anyway.)

Cover this page in things you do well.

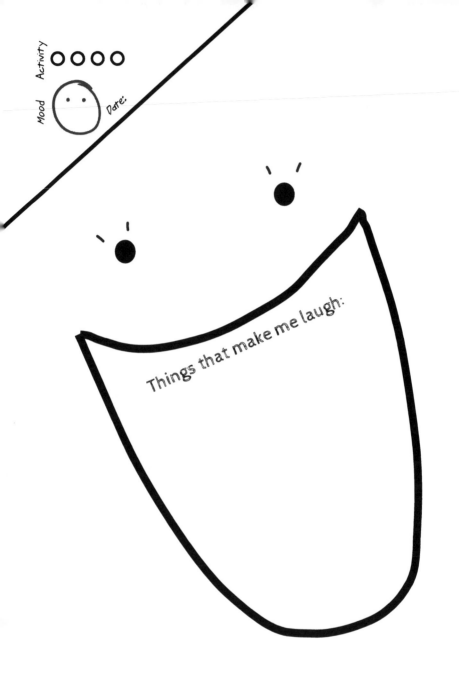

Things that make me laugh:

Some people think laughter
is the best medicine.

61

What makes you `beautiful?´
Cover the page with your wonderful qualities.

Make a wish!

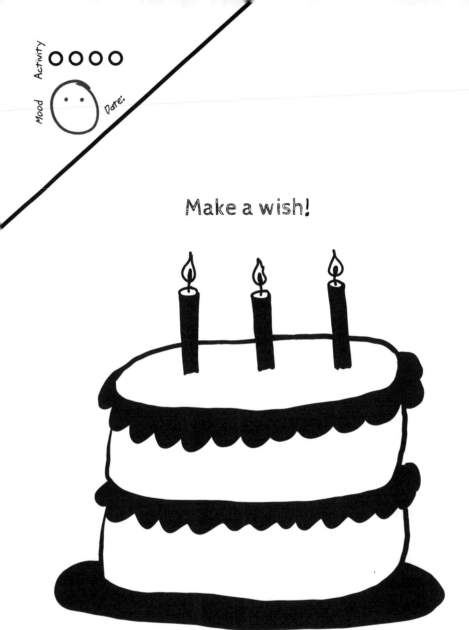

(Even if it's not your birthday.)

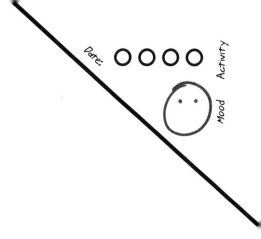
My favorite thing to do with free time is:

_____ .

Runner-up: _____ .

Have you tried to do these things recently?

☐ yes

☐ no

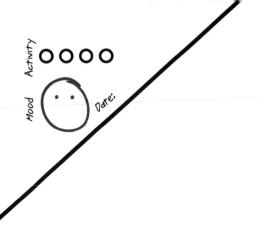

Nice work! You're moving right along in this book.

Maybe your recovery moves at a different pace.
Where do you feel you are on your recovery journey?

Beginning

Middle

End

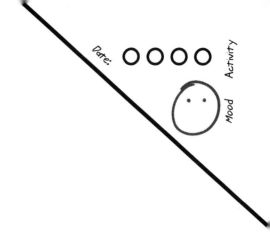
Reflect on your expectations on pages 30, 43, and 44.

How do you feel about your progress so far?

What are your newest expectations?

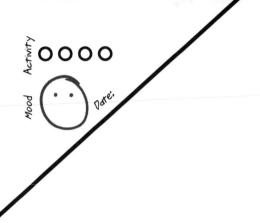

The next section of this book will dig deeper into things that could be holding you back.

Before we start though, let's get motivated. What is a realistic goal for the next week?

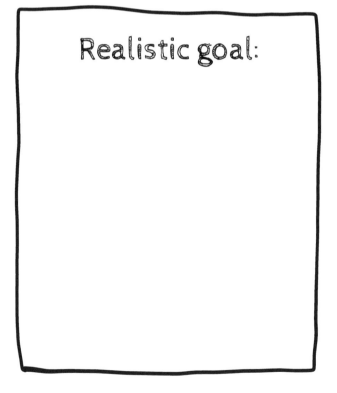

Realistic goal:

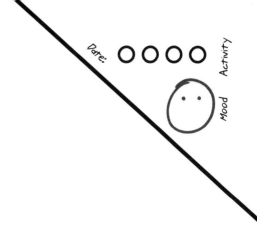
When it comes to this recovery,
I am a teensy bit anxious about:

_____ .

Anxiety can be a good thing.
It's an important part of your intuition.
Recognize it for what it is and nothing more.

Notice when anxiety turns to fear.

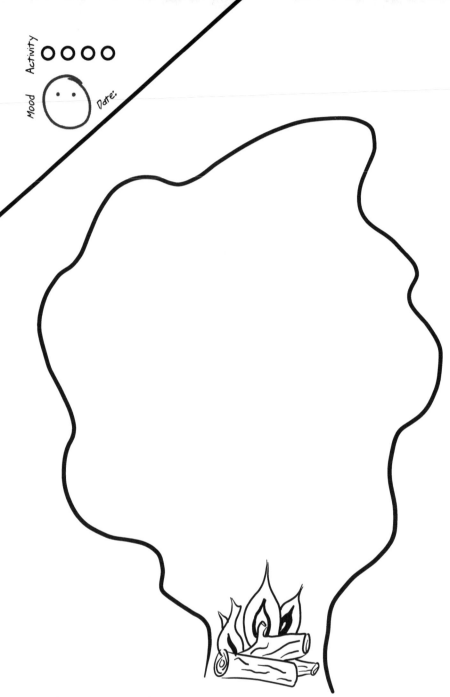

Are you afraid of anything related to your recovery?
Put your fears and worries in the fire.

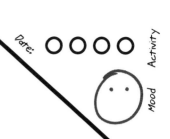
Fear and worry aren't bad things.
In fact, they can be extremely helpful.
They keep us aware of our surroundings. They help us
survive.

Sometimes, though, fear and worry can get in the way.
Too much of them can hold us back.
They can make us think our needs aren't being met.

What do you need most right now?

Can someone on page 31 help you find it?

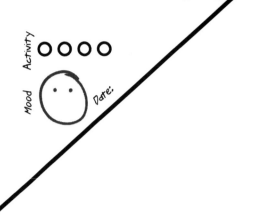

Mood

Activity ○○○○

Date:

Are you covered?

☐ Food

☐ Water

☐ Shelter

☐ Sleep

Let's check in to be sure.

71

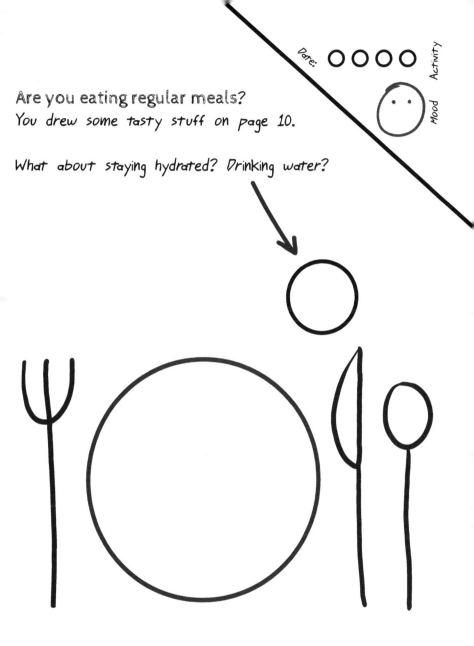

Are you eating regular meals?
You drew some tasty stuff on page 10.

What about staying hydrated? Drinking water?

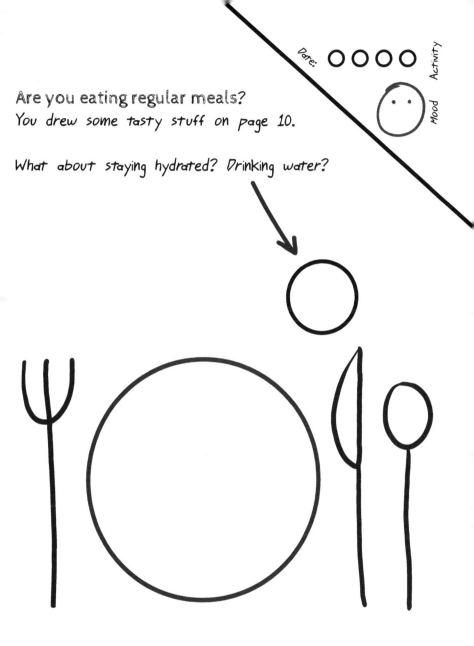

The last thing I ate and drank.

You are what you eat!

Mood   Activity

OOOO

Date:

Rhythms are healing.
Where do you sleep? Is your bed set up for rest and healing?
Take the time to record your sleep for one week, even if you already have
a sense of your patterns. Seeing them written out can be illuminating.

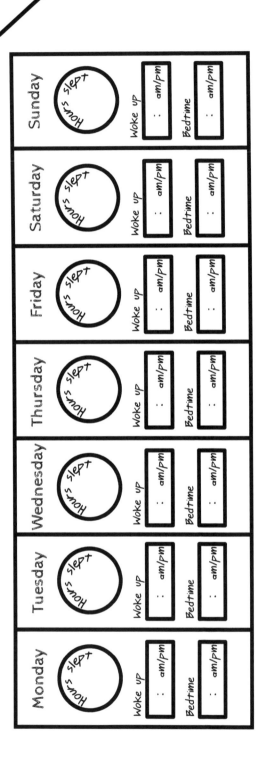

Monday	Tuesday	Wednesday	Thursday	Friday	Saturday	Sunday
Hours slept	Hours slept	Hours slept	Hours slept	Hours slept	Hours slept	Hours slept
Woke up __:__ am/pm	Woke up __:__ am/pm	Woke up __:__ am/pm	Woke up __:__ am/pm	Woke up __:__ am/pm	Woke up __:__ am/pm	Woke up __:__ am/pm
Bedtime __:__ am/pm	Bedtime __:__ am/pm	Bedtime __:__ am/pm	Bedtime __:__ am/pm	Bedtime __:__ am/pm	Bedtime __:__ am/pm	Bedtime __:__ am/pm

What irritates you?

What used to irritate you but doesn't anymore?

Sounds like you are growing!

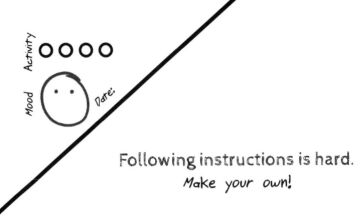

Following instructions is hard.
Make your own!

What my recovery team told me to do	What I did

Remind yourself of the
resources on page 34.

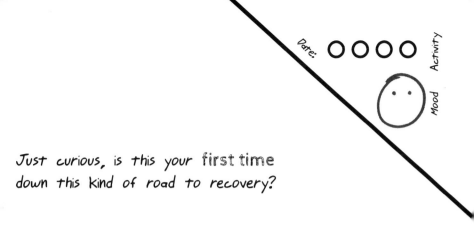

Just curious, is this your first time down this kind of road to recovery?

☐ Yes

☐ No ←

What happened
last time?

Mood Activity

Date:

FULL
RECOVERY

What's standing in the way of your recovery?

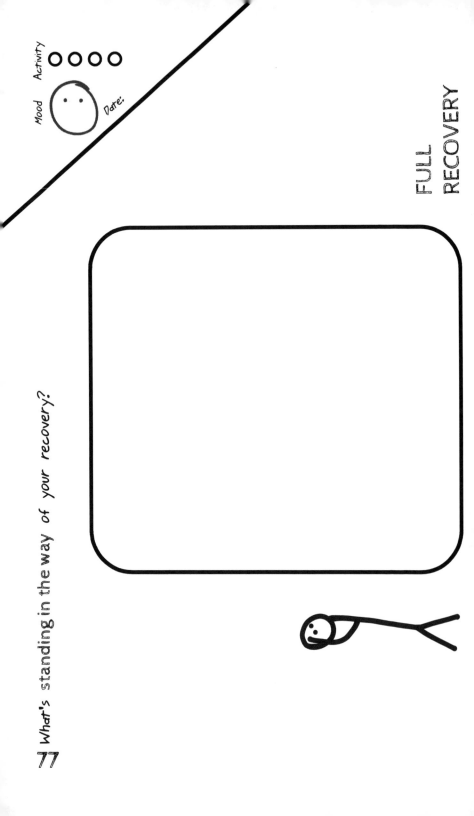

Cover this page in current frustrations.

Then, tear out the page, and enjoy ripping it up.

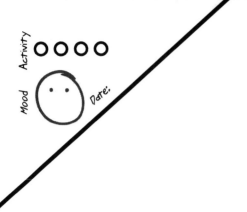

Mood Activity O O O O

Date:

Frustrations be gone!

Date: ⭕⭕⭕⭕

Mood Activity

Check all that apply:

☐ I am capable.

☐ I can do this.

☐ Some people are terrible.

☐ Everything is terrible.

☐ Everything will be okay.

☐ I am strong.

☐ _____

☐ _____

☐ _____

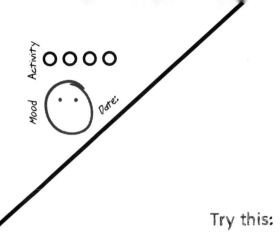

Try this:

Wiggle a tiny part of your body that
you haven't moved in a long time.

Take your time.
Imagine your breath flowing into it.

Body part:

_____

Your body is wise. You can tap into its knowledge.
Focus on parts of your body that have been closed off
for a long time. Explore these parts with kindness.

Sometimes we close off parts of ourselves out of habit or
self-preservation. Open them up gently, and your mind may
follow suit.

Repeat repeat repeat.

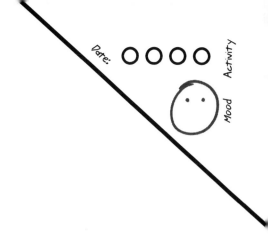

How might your recovery journey
change you for the better?
Check out page 56 for inspiration.

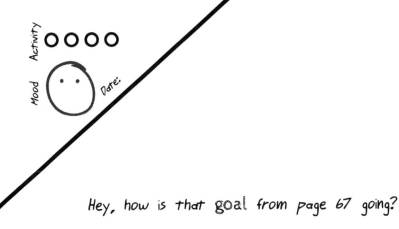

Hey, how is that goal from page 67 going?

Goal progress:

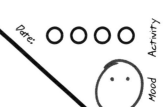

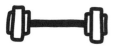

Flip back through your completed activity trackers, and
remind yourself of your tendency on page 16.
See what you can do to be active today.

What helps you keep a healthy activity level?

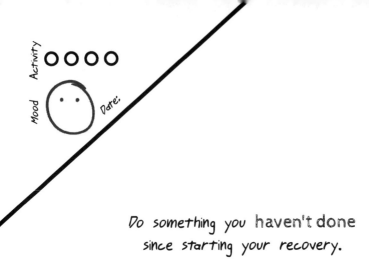

Mood Activity

OOOO

Date:

Do something you haven't done
since starting your recovery.

What did you pick and how did it go?

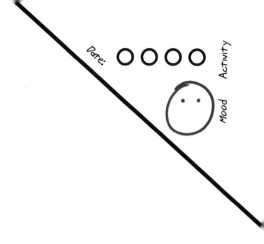

HEALTH
   HEAL
HEAL
 AL
  L

Grow the crossword as much as you can.

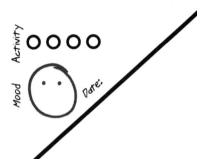

Mood Activity

Date:

Who has really stood out from your recovery team?

What do you like about them?

Acts of service are a good way to stay connected.
Write a letter to a stranger who is starting
a similar recovery tomorrow. Impart your wisdom!

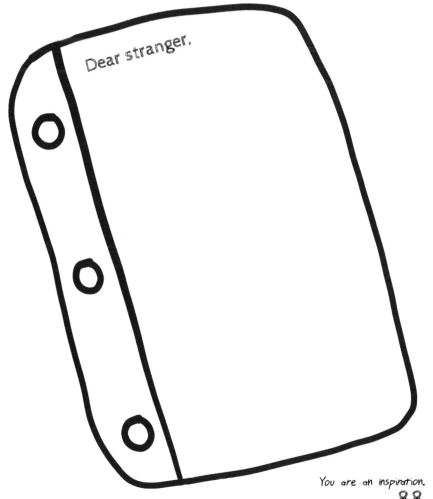

Dear stranger,

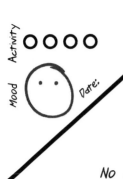

Activity ○ ○ ○ ○

Mood

Date:

No one can set priorities for you.
What would you like to do today?

1)

teeny
tiny
activity

2)

medium
activity

3)

main
activity

Sounds great!
What progress can you make right now?

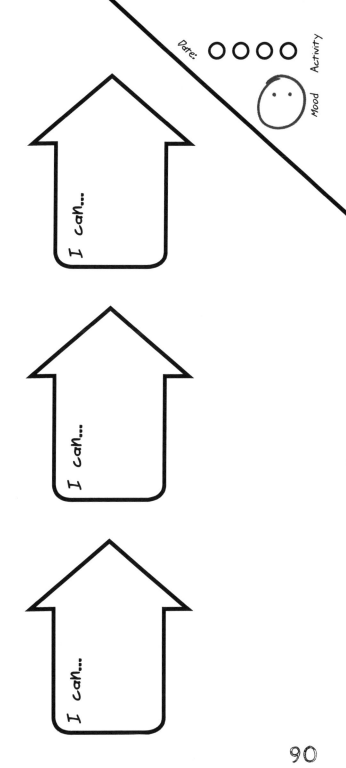

I can...

I can...

I can...

90

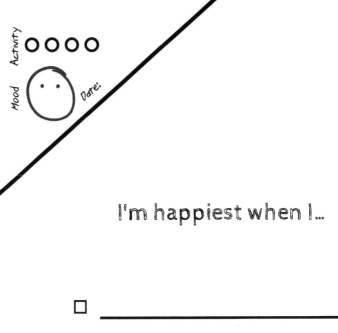

Mood Activity OOOO

Date:

I'm happiest when I...

☐ _____

☐ _____

☐ _____

☐ _____

☐ _____

Pick one item from your list and do it today.

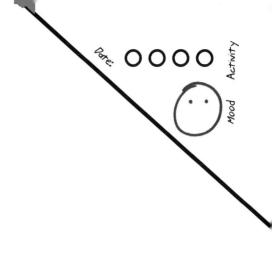
Try this:

Take a moment to stretch
like you just woke up.

Smile imagining the morning sun on your face.

You've just shown you can tap into this feeling anytime!
Use it when you need a boost.
Call on it when you feel lost.
You got this.

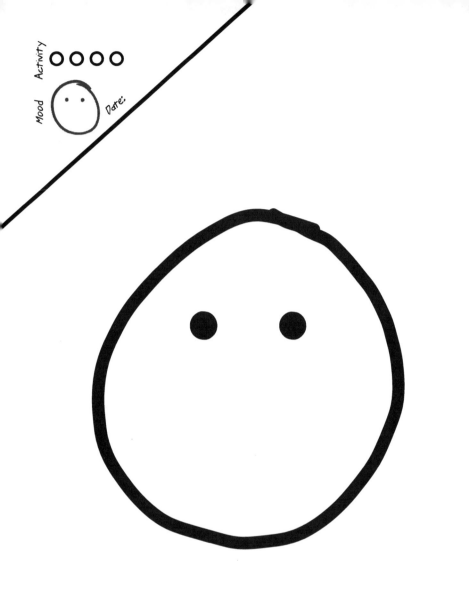

How are the emotions today?
Draw a more detailed face than your typical mood tracker.

93

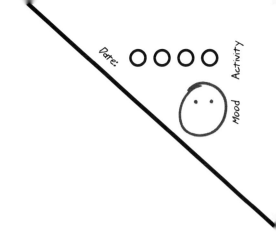

How was a *recent* recovery-related appointment?

Jot a note about it starting on page 197, even if it was a simple get—together, like getting lunch with a friend.

What medications have you been using?

Add them to the list on page 196. Include non—prescription drugs like vitamins and supplements (or anything else you use to self—medicate).

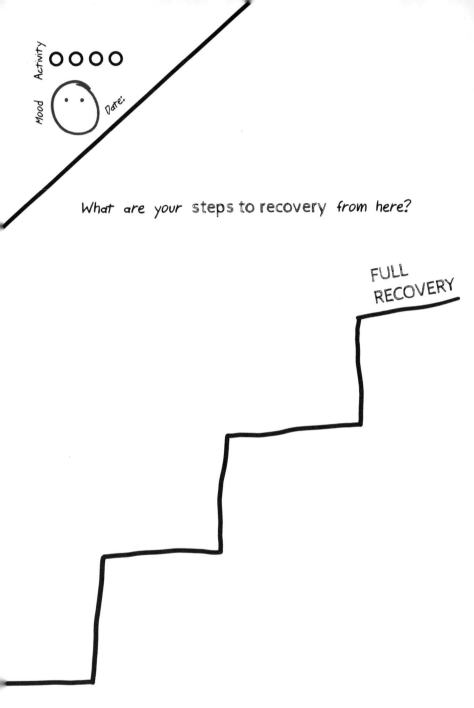

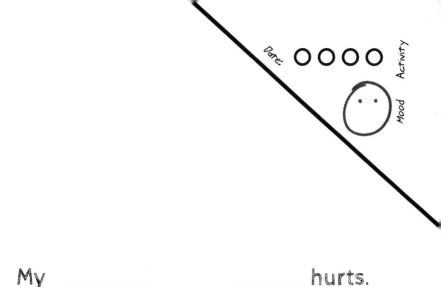

My _____ hurts.

Recovery pain feels different to everyone.
What about you?

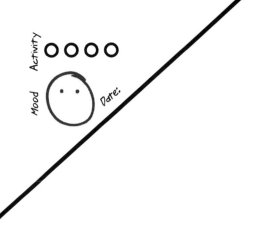

Mood

Activity

O O O O

Date:

What other
people think

Things I can't control

The weather

Cats

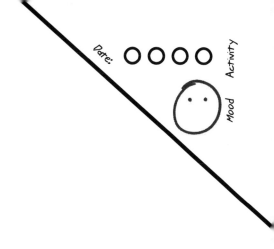

Date: ○ ○ ○ ○

Activity

Mood

Things I can control

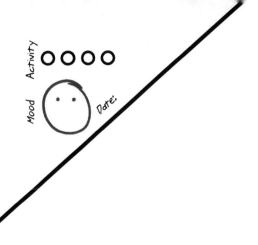

Mood

Activity

○ ○ ○ ○

Date:

Art can be therapeutic.

Color this page, entirely, any way you like.

Are there other kinds of
art you can do today?

99

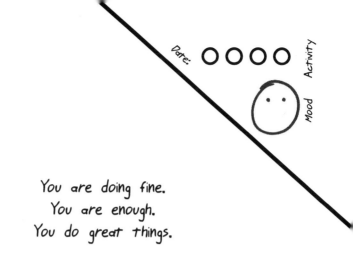

○ ○ ○ ○

You are doing fine.
You are enough.
You do great things.

Draw great things flowing out of you into the world.

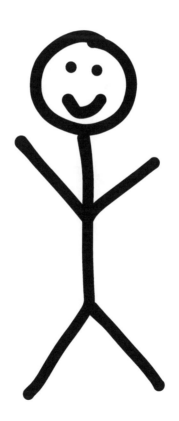

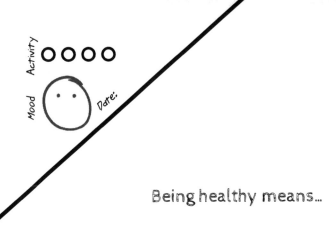

Activity

Mood

Date:

Being healthy means...

It's important to have realistic ideas about this. Nobody is perfect. Remember page 49?

Recovery Report Card

Working in this book at my own pace	A+
Staying positive	
Trying my best	
Setting realistic expectations	
Following recovery instructions	
Connecting with my recovery team	

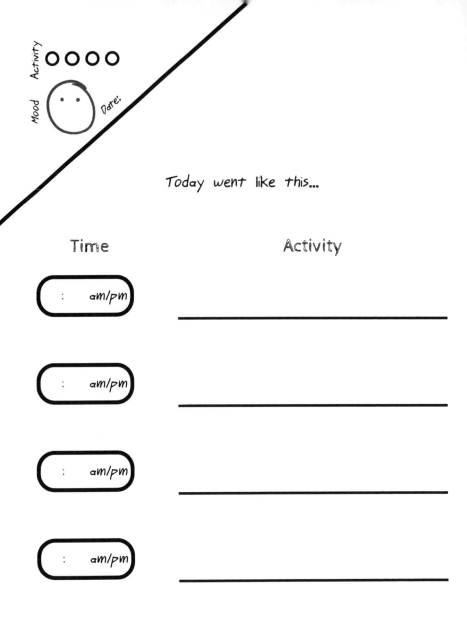

Activity ○○○○

Mood

Date:

Today went like this...

Time

Activity

:   am/pm

_____

:   am/pm

_____

:   am/pm

_____

:   am/pm

_____

Recognizing our habits is an important part of
self-awareness and taking ownership of our lives.
How could tomorrow be the same or different?

Sometimes when you are recovering
you get a lot of unsolicited advice.
All that "help" can get messy
...some of it can be good stuff.

Person	Advice I took

Flip through your mood trackers,
then complete a personal weather forecast:

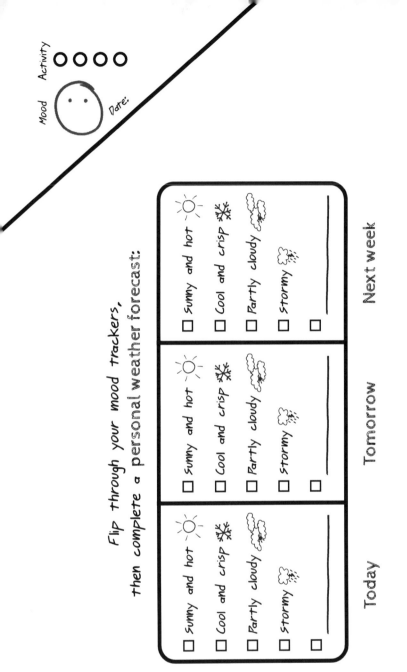

Today

☐ Sunny and hot
☐ Cool and crisp
☐ Partly cloudy
☐ Stormy
☐ _____

Tomorrow

☐ Sunny and hot
☐ Cool and crisp
☐ Partly cloudy
☐ Stormy
☐ _____

Next week

☐ Sunny and hot
☐ Cool and crisp
☐ Partly cloudy
☐ Stormy
☐ _____

Goal for next week:

Great job! You just wrote down a goal.
Did you know you are now more likely to achieve it?

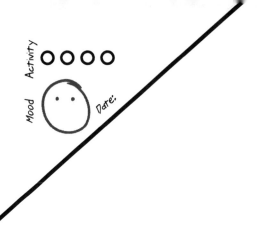

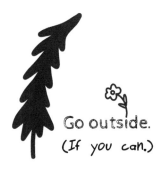

Go outside.
(If you can.)

If you can't get outside, can you get a breath
of fresh air through a window or door?

107

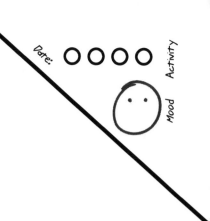

Date: ○○○○

Mood

Activity

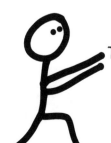

Today I pushed myself by...

108

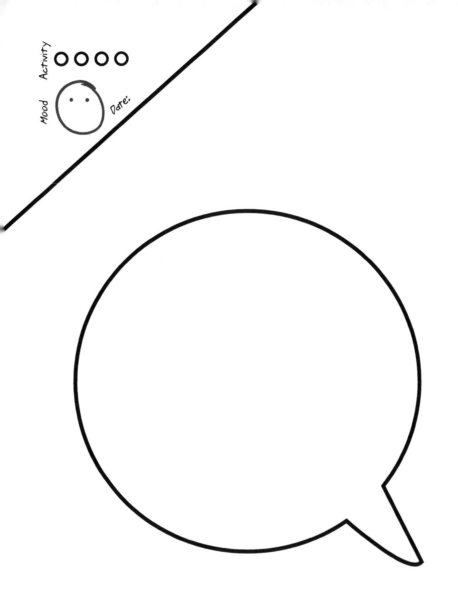

Who is your role model?
What would they say to you today?

You're well into your recovery now. Give yourself a pat on the back:

Certificate of Achievement

TO:

For outstanding progress, specifically:

On this ____ day of ____ in the year ____ .

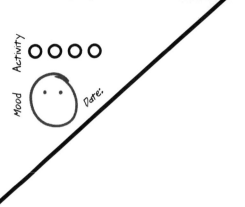

Ask someone from your recovery team for an honest assessment of your progress so far.

What did they have to say?

Do you agree with them?

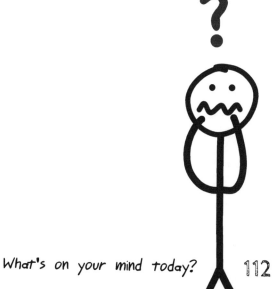

What's on your mind today?

112

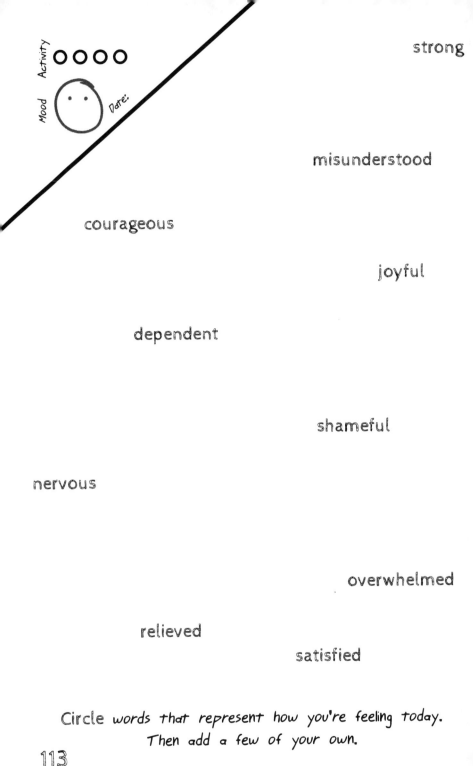

Mood Activity

○ ○ ○ ○

Date:

strong

misunderstood

courageous

joyful

dependent

shameful

nervous

overwhelmed

relieved

satisfied

Circle words that represent how you're feeling today.
Then add a few of your own.

113

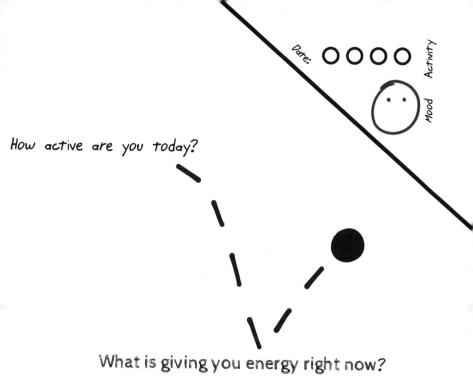

Date: ○ ○ ○ ○

Mood   Activity

How active are you today?

What is giving you energy right now?

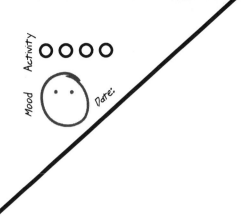

Mood Activity Date:

Sometimes recovery journeys make people angry.
Yell it out here in ALL CAPITALS.

This is one of many methods to release anger.
Whatever method you choose, make sure you build yourself
an emotion release valve.

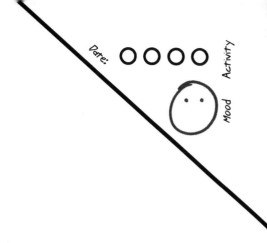

Three ways to calm down when I'm triggered:

1

2

3

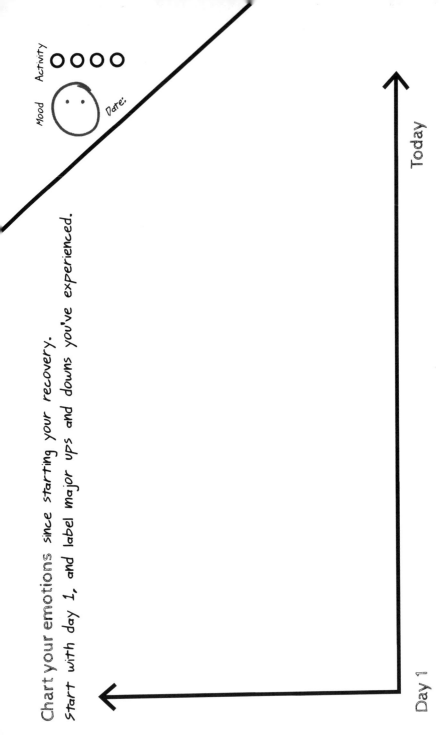

Chart your emotions since starting your recovery. Start with day 1, and label major ups and downs you've experienced.

Mood   Activity

Date:

Today

Day 1

117

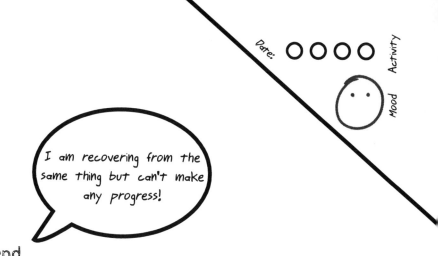

Friend

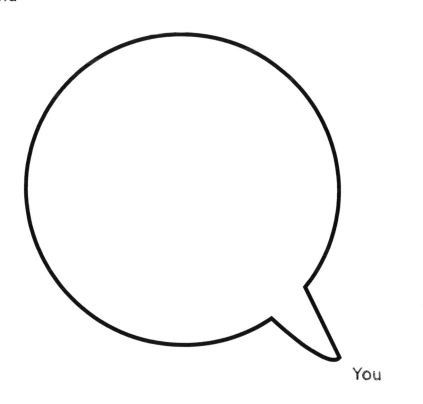

You

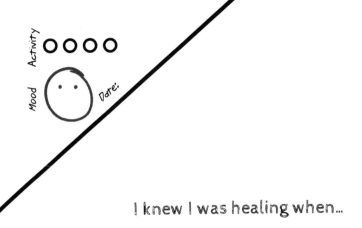

Mood Activity Date:

I knew I was healing when...

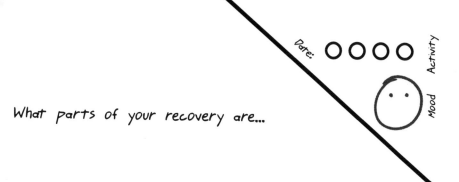

What parts of your recovery are...

Encouraging

✛✛
─ ─

Discouraging

Now rip out the discouraging half, tear it up,
and let's move on.

120

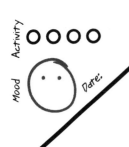

Mood Activity

Date:

Have there been any **surprises** during your recovery?

What was out of the ordinary or **unexpected**? How did you handle it?

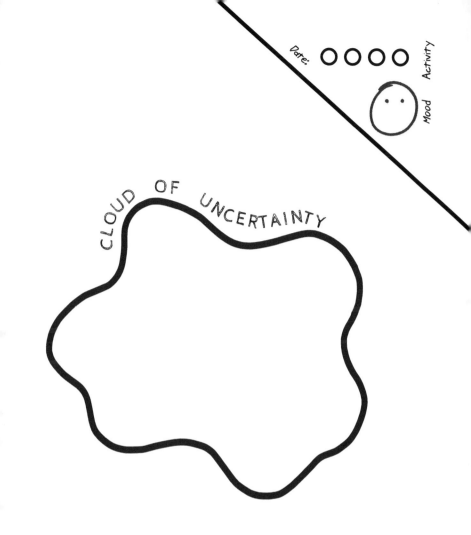

CLOUD OF UNCERTAINTY

This cloud can be annoying. It can show up in response to unexpected changes in plans or progress.

But clouds are flexible, like you. You can adjust your expectations to fit new circumstances.

What's in your cloud of uncertainty?

122

Mood Activity ○ ○ ○ ○

Date:

I can _____

I can _____

I can _____

I can _____

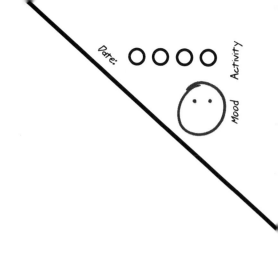
Sometimes when we're healing we spend a lot of time in one spot. Even so, we're not always aware of our surroundings.

Draw something here that you see every day (your room, chair, window, etc.). Take your time. Include details you haven't noticed before.

Build focus.
124

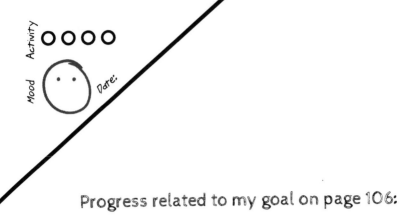

Mood Activity

Date:

Progress related to my goal on page 106:

It's okay to revise your goal if you need to,
but don't give up on it!

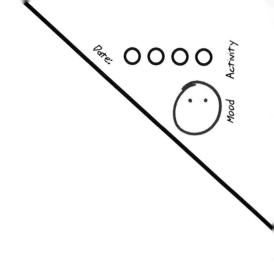

This recovery is…
(Check all that apply.)

- ☐ someone else's fault.
- ☐ bad luck.
- ☐ unexpected.
- ☐ the result of my behavior.
- ☐ what makes me who I am.
- ☐ manageable.
- ☐ a lesson.
- ☐ part of a larger process.
- ☐ _____
- ☐ _____
- ☐ _____

What does your self-talk sound like these days?

We are our own worst critic.
If you wrote down anything hurtful, cross it out.

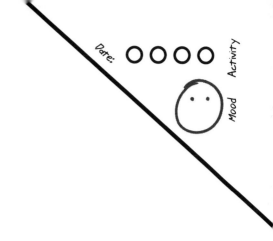
Let's do a body scan.

Get comfortable.
Then, place your attention in each toe, one by one.
(Give each toe at least a minute of attention.)

What do you notice?

Then turn the page
128

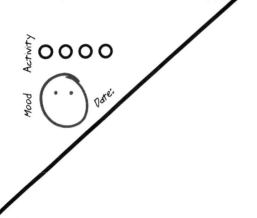

Now slowly and intentionally move your attention up your body. Breathe into every nook and cranny, every fold, every vertebrae. Don't try to fix anything. Don't judge. Just see how things feel. Take several minutes to go all the way to the top of your head.

What did you find? Do any places feel "off-limits"?

This exercise can help connect emotions to parts of the body. The connections offer clues into how we might store past experience in our bodies (like on page 81).

Places that are difficult to feel are often full of powerful potential. Keep them in mind as you are healing.

Open sesame!

Recovery BINGO

Positive self-talk	Sipped fresh air	Healthy lunch	6+ hours sleep last night	Wrote down a goal
Called a friend	Did something just for fun	Left the house	Tried something new	Recognized negative thoughts
Healthy breakfast	Left comfort zone	FREE	Showered	Performed random act of kindness
Made some art	Got dressed	Positive attitude	Reached a goal	Healthy dinner
Completed 5 pages in this book	Exercised	6 glasses of water today	High-fived someone	Laughed

Can you get BINGO this week?

Seriously, try to get five in a row.

It's been [ ] ish days since I started my recovery.

Things are:

☐ right on track.

☐ a little slow.

☐ faster than I expected.

☐ not going well.

☐ an adventure.

☐ _____ .

Because:

131

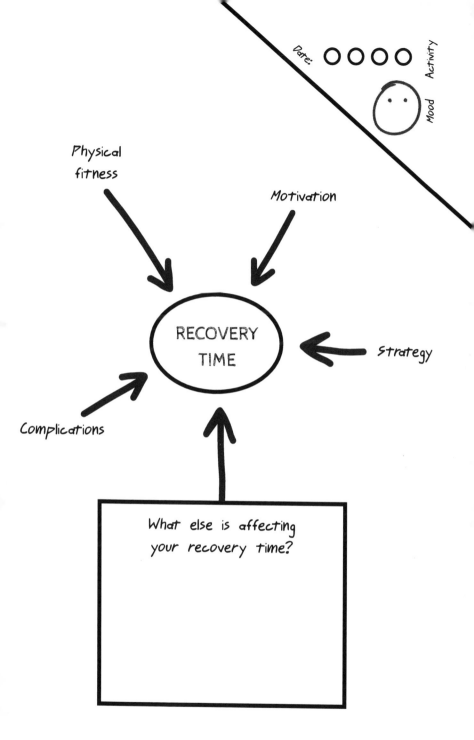

Physical
fitness

Motivation

RECOVERY
TIME

Strategy

Complications

What else is affecting
your recovery time?

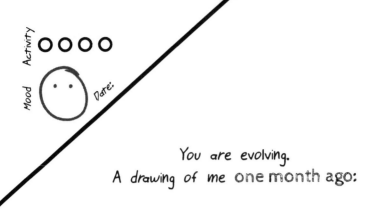

Mood Activity

O O O O

Date:

You are evolving.
A drawing of me one month ago:

A drawing of me today:

Are you sporting any new gear?

133

Has your recovery impacted your senses?
Mark the scales to show any changes.

sight   less sensitive ———————— same ———————— more sensitive

smell   less sensitive ———————— same ———————— more sensitive

taste   less sensitive ———————— same ———————— more sensitive

touch   less sensitive ———————— same ———————— more sensitive

hearing   less sensitive ———————— same ———————— more sensitive

intuition   less sensitive ———————— same ———————— more sensitive

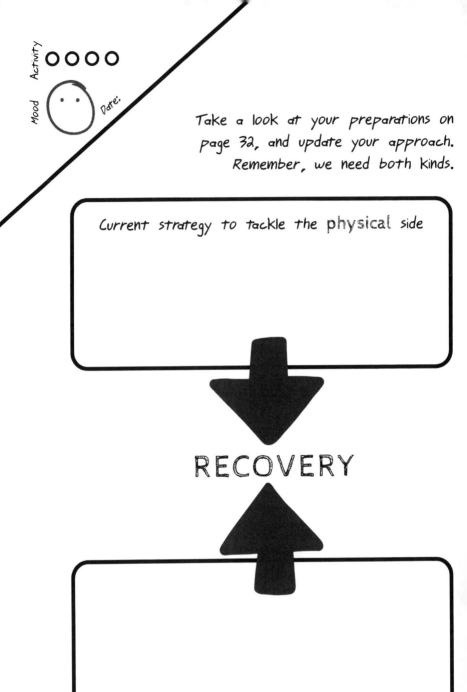

Take a look at your preparations on page 32, and update your approach. Remember, we need both kinds.

Current strategy to tackle the physical side

RECOVERY

Current strategy to tackle the mental side

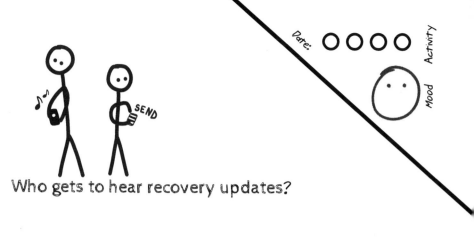

Who gets to hear recovery updates?

What kinds of updates do you keep to yourself?

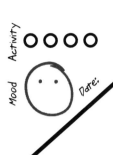

Mood Activity

Date:

Three ways I regularly engage my recovery team:
For data, see page 197.

1)

2)

3)

Gratitude never hurts. *Here's a thank you note to get you started. (You could even deliver it.)*

Dear _____,

My recovery has been _____

THANK YOU

for all you've done to help me through it, especially _____

With gratitude, _____

138

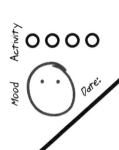

Complete the word search:

E	A	P	R	A	C	T	I	C	A	L	A
L	P	A	P	H	S	S	L	E	A	E	L
Y	H	T	L	A	E	H	O	C	H	O	S
O	A	I	E	P	L	A	H	P	P	C	A
U	Y	E	A	P	R	O	G	R	E	S	S
L	A	N	A	Y	E	K	S	E	R	L	L
U	L	C	T	I	A	L	I	H	E	A	E
N	R	E	C	O	V	E	R	N	A	L	E
K	L	L	E	N	R	A	S	S	D	R	P
S	R	O	N	I	G	R	M	L	A	C	V
E	S	O	V	I	C	A	M	I	E	L	W
P	A	S	W	E	N	C	T	N	E	A	I

kind	progress	recover
work	patience	love
happy	healthy	calm
sleep	you	practical

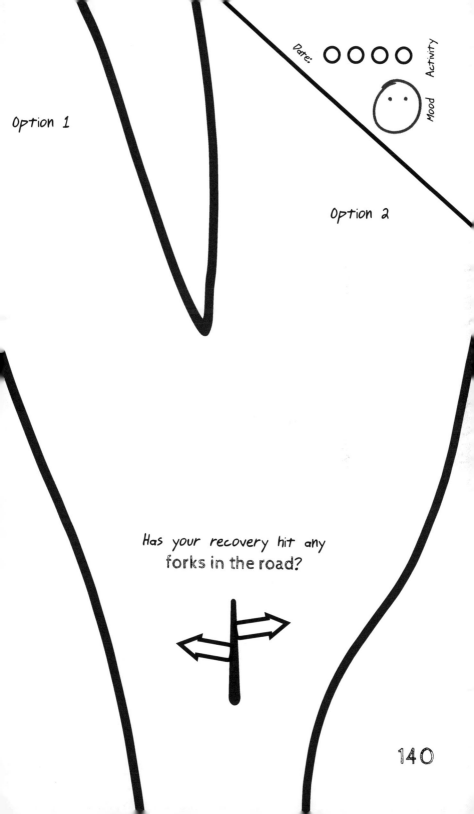

Option 1

Activity

Mood

Option 2

Has your recovery hit any
forks in the road?

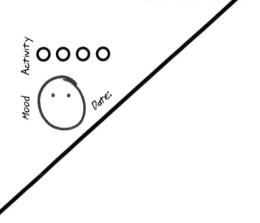

Mood

Activity

Date:

What was simple about today?

What was complicated about today?

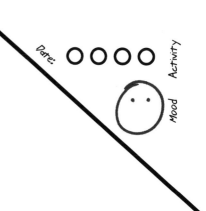
Today I am:
(Circle one)

an optimist

a pessimist

a realist

_____

know thyself.

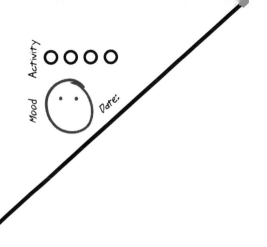

It's okay for me to let _____ go,

so I can heal.

Recovery takes a lot of energy.
However you got here, you are 143 pages in! You may be
starting to take on more responsibilities or be feeling more
capable than ever. Or not. Either way, you have to let
some tasks go while you heal. Prioritize.

143

...and go easy on yourself!

Have fun covering this page in soothing squiggles.

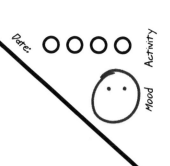

Date:

Mood

Activity

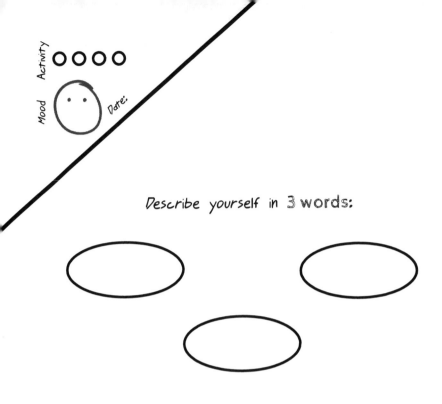
Describe yourself in 3 words:

Ask someone else to do the same:

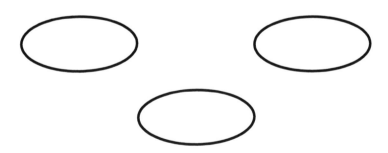

Do you see what they see?

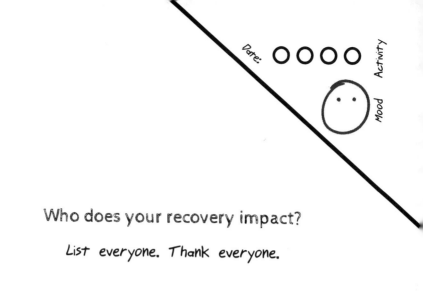

Who does your recovery impact?

List everyone. Thank everyone.

Gratitude does more than foster compassion. Many studies have connected feelings of gratitude to improved sleep, energy, health, and healing. Gratitude also helps keep us connected to support systems and the world around us.

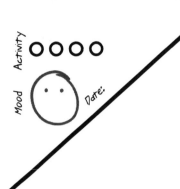

What questions remain about your recovery?

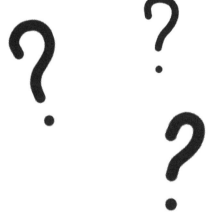

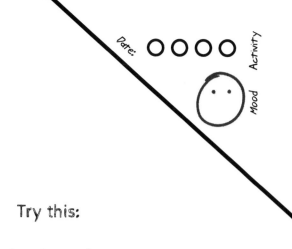

Try this:

Sit comfortably and quietly.
Imagine a peaceful scene.

Keep adding detail to the image in your mind.
Make it vivid. Make it comprehensive.
Only add things to the scene that you find beautiful.

Enjoy the time thinking about it.
That's it.

Moments like this can flush us with positive brain chemicals that help us heal. It's a proven strategy to help cultivate a positive mental attitude.

(That comes in handy no matter the situation.)

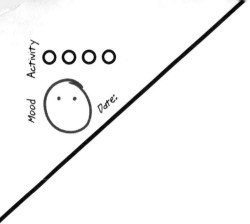
Have you been avoiding any parts of your recovery?

Cross out any avoidance strategies below that resonate with you. Add any that are missing. Cross those out, too. Allow this to be a symbolic, first step away from these strategies.

Social media	Stay indoors	Complain to friends	
Sleep	Withdraw from friends and family		

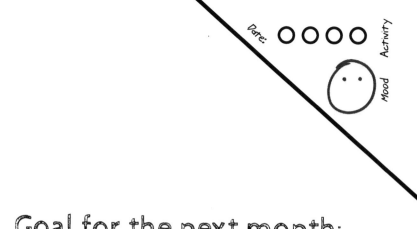

Goal for the next month:

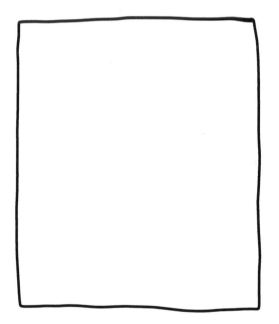

Fill the balloons with things that keep your spirits high.

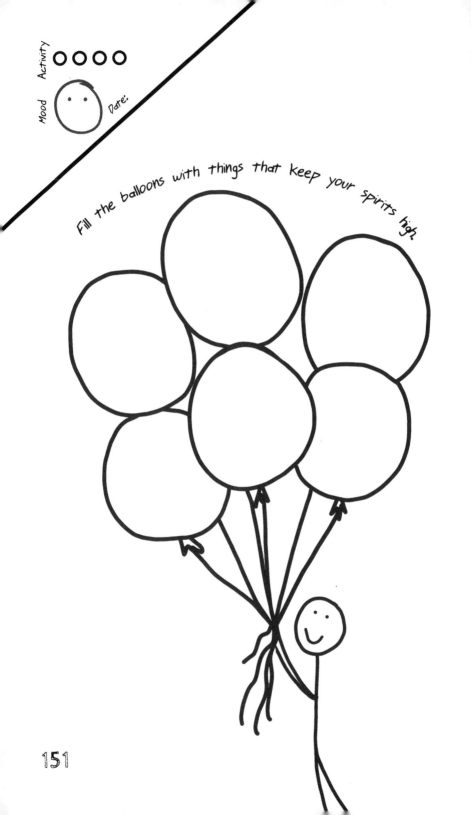

151

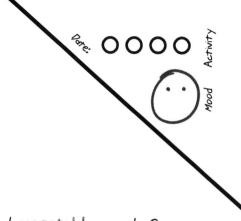

Date: ○ ○ ○ ○

Mood

Activity

Did you eat fruits and vegetables today?

☐ Yes
I ate:

☐ No
I ate:

152

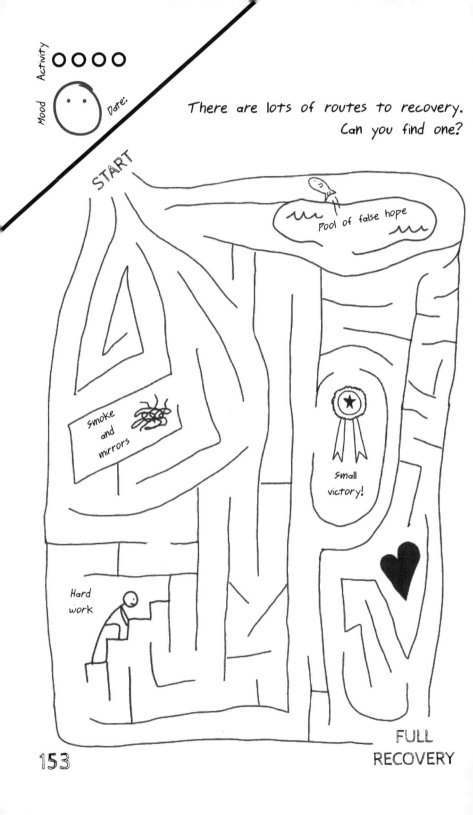

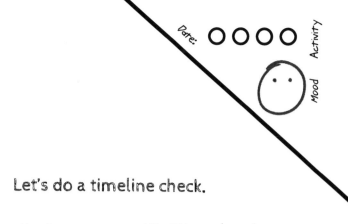

Let's do a timeline check.

Check out the timeline on pages 43–44, and update your vision for the future here.

	I'll probably feel...	I'll probably be able to...
in 1 week		
in 1 month		
in 1 year		

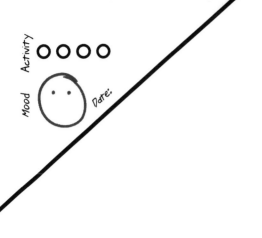

Mood

Activity

Date:

I can't wait to _____

when I'm fully recovered!

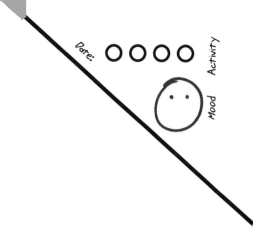

Go back to those self portraits you drew
on pages 6 and 133.

How has your self-image changed?

How you see yourself is directly related to
how others see you. Love yourself and others
can love you. Positive self-image creates a
positive feedback loop for everyone.

156

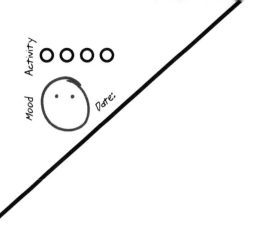

Support systems are critical. They are two-way streets. How do you contribute to the most important relationships in your life?

Important relationship	Recent effort to strengthen relationship

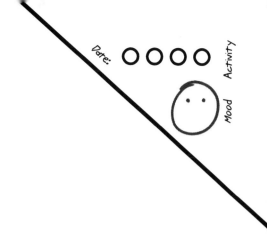
When is the last time you had an appointment
related to your recovery?

Check out your appointment log on page 197.
Are you due for a check-in with someone?
Schedule it now.

Date:

Today I feel _____ .

I'll probably spend most of the day

_____ .

If it proves to be too _____ ,

I'll _____ instead.

Be honest. Make a plan.

159

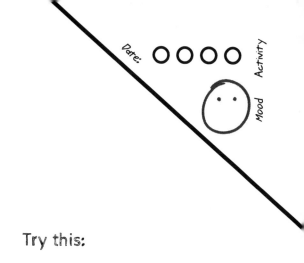

Try this:

Go breathe in a scent that you like.

Smell can uplift. A good smell can leave us smiling and freshly motivated. Our sense of smell is also tied closely to memory. It can bring up past experiences that might guide us in the present.

Did any memories come to mind?

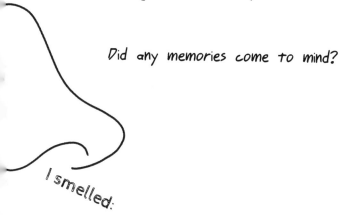

I smelled:

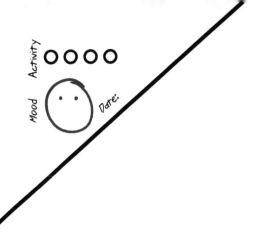

Mood Activity

Date:

Repeat page 107.

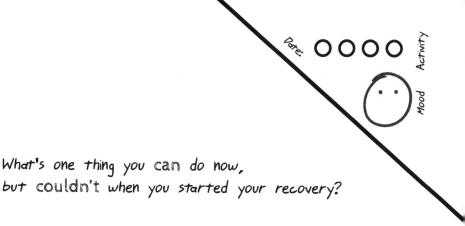

What's one thing you can do now,
but couldn't when you started your recovery?

How did it feel when you did it for the first time?

It's important to recognize progress, however large or
small. Looking back reminds us how far we've come.
The road ahead may be long, but so is the road you've
already traveled!

162

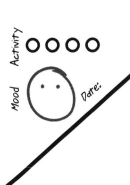

Mood Activity

Date:

3 things to help answer questions on page 147:

1)

2)

3)

163

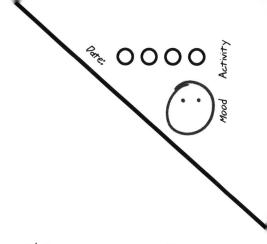

What good things could happen tomorrow?

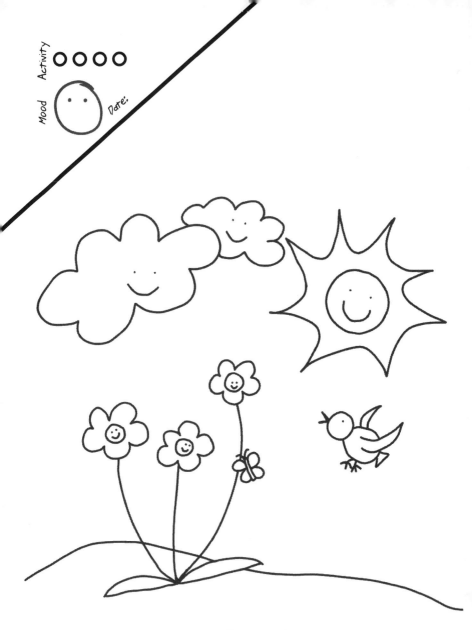

Be angry all over this scene.

Check in with your body. See how it feels to go from happy to angry in one page. What do you notice?

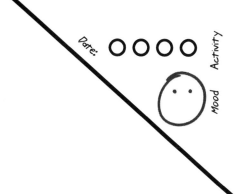
Emotions are noisy.
That's why they keep showing up in this book!

Emotions can be a good thing, as you well know.
They help us recognize and let go of things we cling to.
Emotions need to be expressed. That's the only way to
process them. If we keep them stored in our bodies, they
can overwhelm the healing process.

Describe a time when emotions took over your recovery.

Connect emotions to your
body on page 128.

166

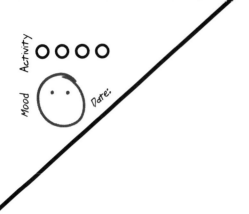

When emotional thoughts sneak into your mind,
are they mostly about the:

past

present

future

Recognize your patterns.

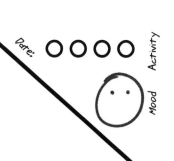

Let's see how the past compares to the present.
Place a mark at the appropriate spot on each line.

When I filled out page 29, I felt:

0 |-----------------------------| 100%

Today I feel:

0 |-----------------------------| 100%

While the past offers context, try to face forward.
Let the future unfold in new ways.

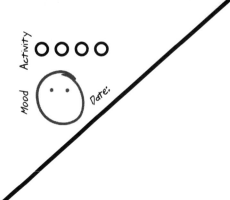

My warning flags to avoid this whole thing
in the future:

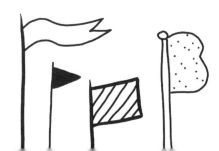

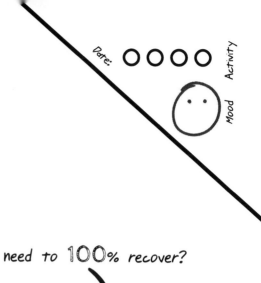

What is something else you need to 100% recover?

How will you get it?

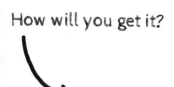

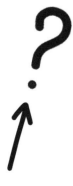

170

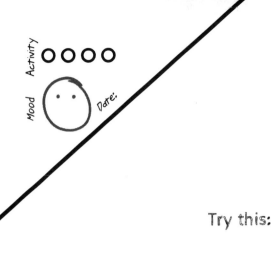

Try this:

Turn on some of your favorite music.
If you can't turn on music,
hear a tune in your head.

Close your eyes.

Focus only on the music and your breathing.

Music has healing properties.
(It's a different kind of art therapy.)
A simple tune can improve a person's mood.
Music has also been shown to help people heal faster.
Enjoy this powerful approach.

Turn it up!

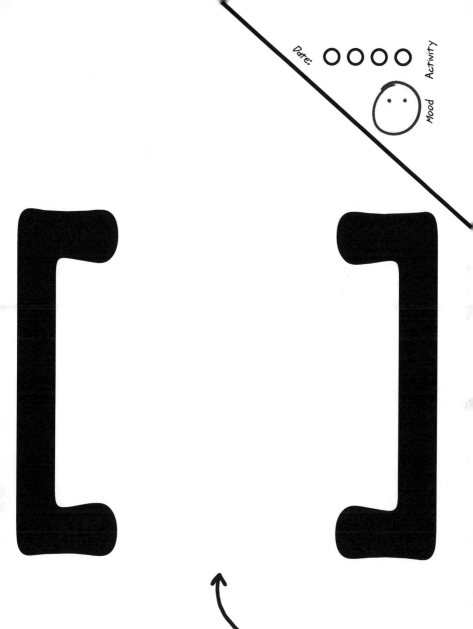

[   ]

Do a brain dump.
Jot down your most
recurrent thoughts here.

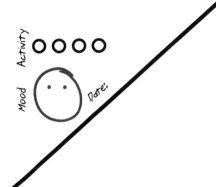
Lest we forget, experts agree managing expectations is a critical part of recovery.
We can guess, but we never know what will happen.
Go back to the two possible outcomes you described on page 37 and 38.

What in between thing actually happened?

What else did you expect to happen?

Turn to Pages 30, 43 and 44 for inspiration.

Has it happened?

☐ yes ☐ no

☐ yes ☐ no

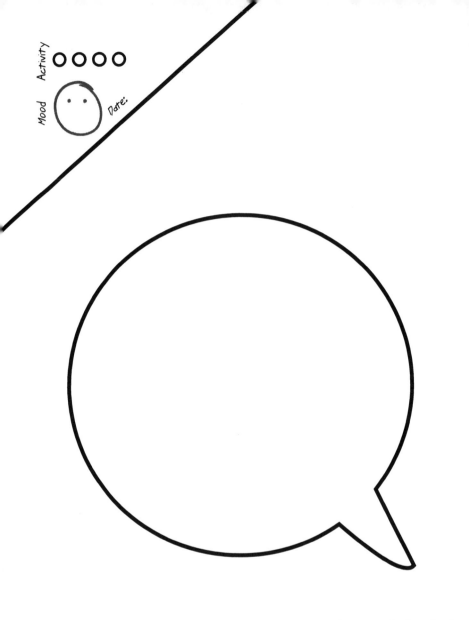

How have you learned to ask for help
since starting your recovery?
Be specific.

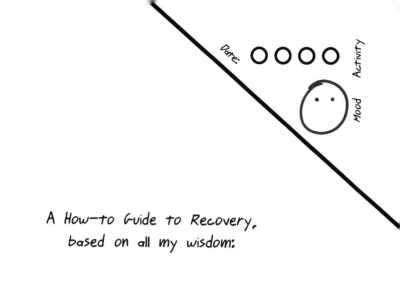

Activity

Mood

A How—to Guide to Recovery,
based on all my wisdom:

step 1:

step 2:

step 3:

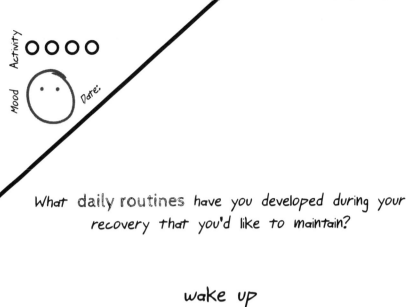

What daily routines have you developed during your recovery that you'd like to maintain?

<u>wake up</u>

_____

_____

_____

_____

_____

<u>go to bed</u>

Look ahead. What can you do over the next year to support:

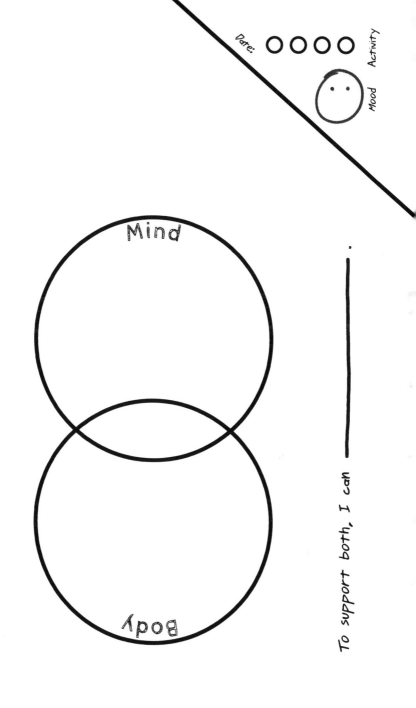

Mind

Body

To support both, I can _____.

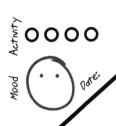

Mood

Activity

Date:

This book has told you to do a lot of things.
Do what you need, all over these two pages.
Writing and drawing can bring clarity.
This time, try it on your own.

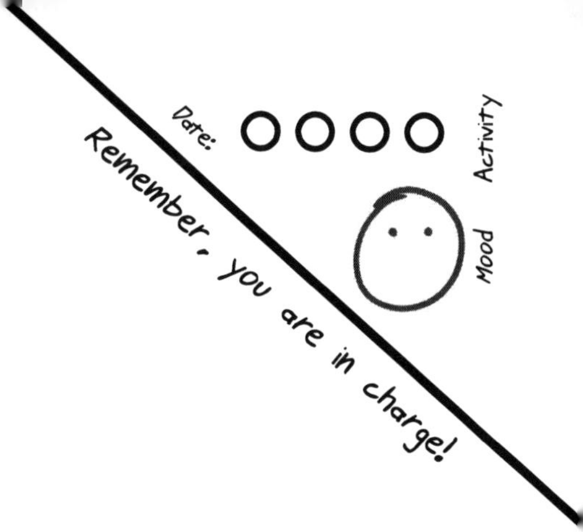

Date: ○○○○

Remember, you are in charge!

Mood

Activity

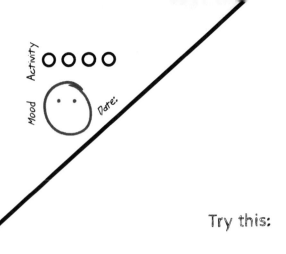

Mood Activity

Date:

Try this:

Close your eyes.
Focus on your breath.
Say a mental "in" and "out" with each one.

Start with a set of three breaths.

Repeat.
Make space.

This approach, and all the others in this book, are always available to you. You can call on them any time.

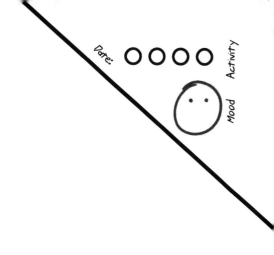

Date:

Mood

Activity

Now, with a calm mind, let's begin to reflect on your recovery so far.

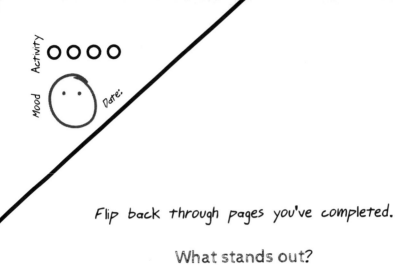

Mood Activity

O O O O

Date:

Flip back through pages you've completed.

What stands out?

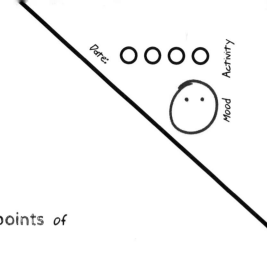
What have been the high points of
your recovery so far?

What have been the low points?

The end is in sight,
but that's just this book.

184

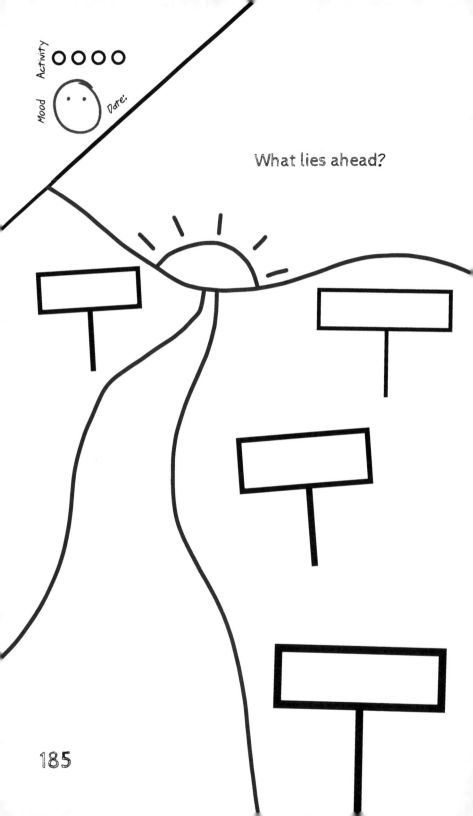

What lies ahead?

What have you learned from this process?

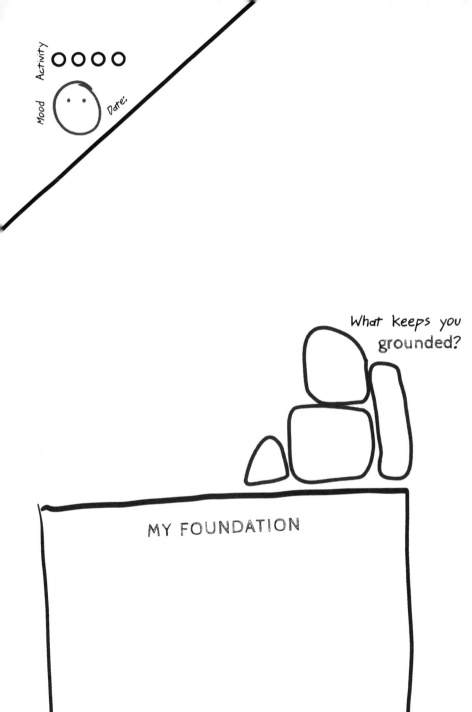

Mood

Activity ○ ○ ○ ○

Date:

What keeps you grounded?

MY FOUNDATION

187

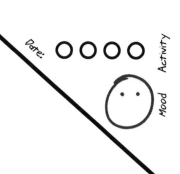

Date: ⭕⭕⭕⭕

Mood   Activity

Resources for after this book is complete:

My friend, _____

My favorite motivator, _____

My activity buddy, _____

This book

And of course, _____

Check out page 34 for more.

188

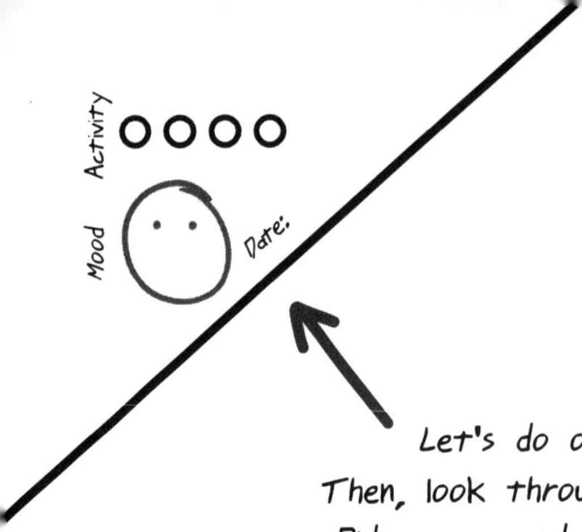

Mood Activity

○ ○ ○ ○

Date:

Let's do one more tracker.
Then, look through your past trackers.
Did you record your mood or activity
level? Why or why not?

How can you maintain recovery momentum?

You can revisit pages from this book again and again until your recovery is complete. Repeat pages, compare pages, and be proud of your progress.

All you need is a paper and pen
(...and sometimes not even that).

Review the progress you've made already
on pages 90, 111, and 162.

What are you most proud of?

What else is important to include
about this experience?

Thank you for sharing
so much of yourself.
192

You made it! Way to go!

Just because this book is ending, doesn't mean your recovery is, or has to.
(It might be just beginning.)

Consider this book a launching pad.
Reflect on what you've shared here.
Tell your friends. Throw a party. Celebrate!

You deserve it.

And one more page before you go...

Dear Recovered Self,

With love,

Tear out the letter on the previous page and put it in
a safe place. (Write on both sides if needed.)
May it provide long—term encouragement and inspiration
as you move forward.

195

MEDICATION LOG

Medicine:

Looks like

Dose: Frequency:

Why:

Makes me feel:

Medicine:

Looks like

Dose: Frequency:

Why:

Makes me feel:

Medicine:

Looks like

Dose: Frequency:

Why:

Makes me feel:

Medicine:

Looks like

Dose: Frequency:

Why:

Makes me feel:

Medicine:

Looks like

Dose: Frequency:

Why:

Makes me feel:

Medicine:

Looks like

Dose: Frequency:

Why:

Makes me feel:

APPOINTMENT LOG

Date

Time

: am/pm

Met with:

Where:

How'd it go?

Date

Time

: am/pm

Met with:

Where:

How'd it go?

Date

Time

: am/pm

Met with:

Where:

How'd it go?

Date

Time

: am/pm

Met with:

Where:

How'd it go?

197

Date

Time
: am/pm

Met with:

Where:

How'd it go?

Date

Time
: am/pm

Met with:

Where:

How'd it go?

Date

Time
: am/pm

Met with:

Where:

How'd it go?

Date

Time
: am/pm

Met with:

Where:

How'd it go?

APPOINTMENT LOG

Date

Time

:   am/pm

Met with:

Where:

How'd it go?

Date

Time

:   am/pm

Met with:

Where:

How'd it go?

Date

Time

:   am/pm

Met with:

Where:

How'd it go?

Date

Time

:   am/pm

Met with:

Where:

How'd it go?

Date

Time

: am/pm

Met with:

Where:

How'd it go?

Date

Time

: am/pm

Met with:

Where:

How'd it go?

Date

Time

: am/pm

Met with:

Where:

How'd it go?

Date

Time

: am/pm

Met with:

Where:

How'd it go?

Made in the USA
Middletown, DE
09 August 2022

70863290R00125